Juice for Health

Juice Fasting for Health and Wellness

by Jennifer Wells

Table of Contents

Resources

Additional works by Jennifer Wells:

Going Gluten Free:
A Quick Start Guide for a Gluten-Free Diet

Top 10 Tips to Help You Lose Weight

Introduction

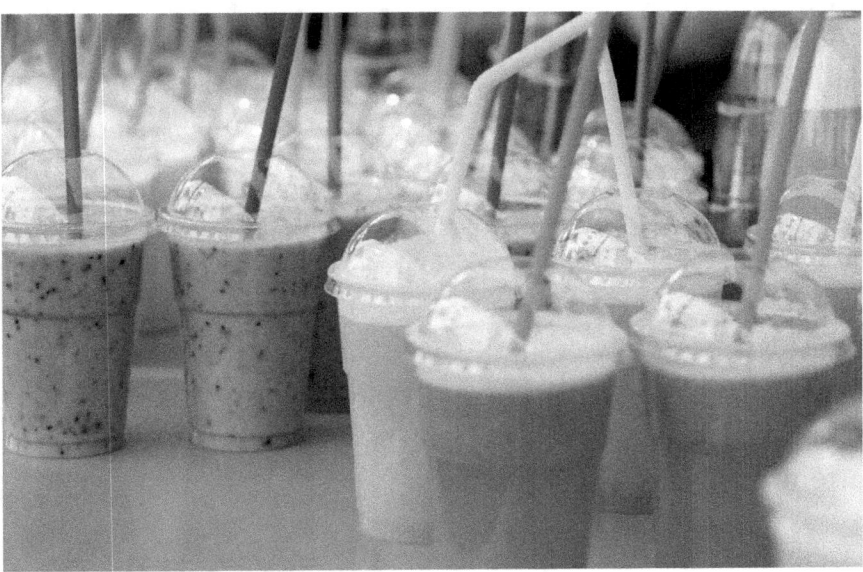

While juices have often been used for medicinal purposes, dating as far back as biblical times,[1] juicing is an area of health I didn't have much personal experience with until a few years ago. Nowadays, when people speak about juicing, it is often in the context of only drinking juices for several days or weeks at a time. Seldom will you ever hear people refer to juicing as a beverage they made to drink with their breakfast. Instead, juicing is practiced as a way to detox one's body of toxins, as well as a way to enjoy health benefits and weight loss. For the purposes of this book, we will speak of juicing as a way to nourish the body for some extended period of time.

At that time, I came across some information that personally challenged me to attempt a juice fast. I wanted to experience firsthand and better understand how it would affect me physically as well as how I would handle this effort on an emotional level.

As I did some in-depth research, I made some decisions concerning how long I would do a juice fast, what combinations of fruits and vegetables I would try, and things I would do and not do. My journey has been a personal one that I will share with you throughout the pages of this book. At the same time, I want to give you helpful information that will empower you so you can decide for yourself if you want to attempt juicing—whether you choose to enjoy juicing occasionally or desire to attempt a fast on a regular basis.

We will explore some positives and negatives concerning juicing, as well as discuss ways to start and end a fast. While some of the material presented here may sound too "formal" or informational, it is because I don't want to sway you one way or the other. What I experience when I juice may not be what happens for you at all, however, I do want you to have a personal viewpoint into this area of health.

With that said, I now take you into the world of juicing!

What is Juicing and How Do I Do It?

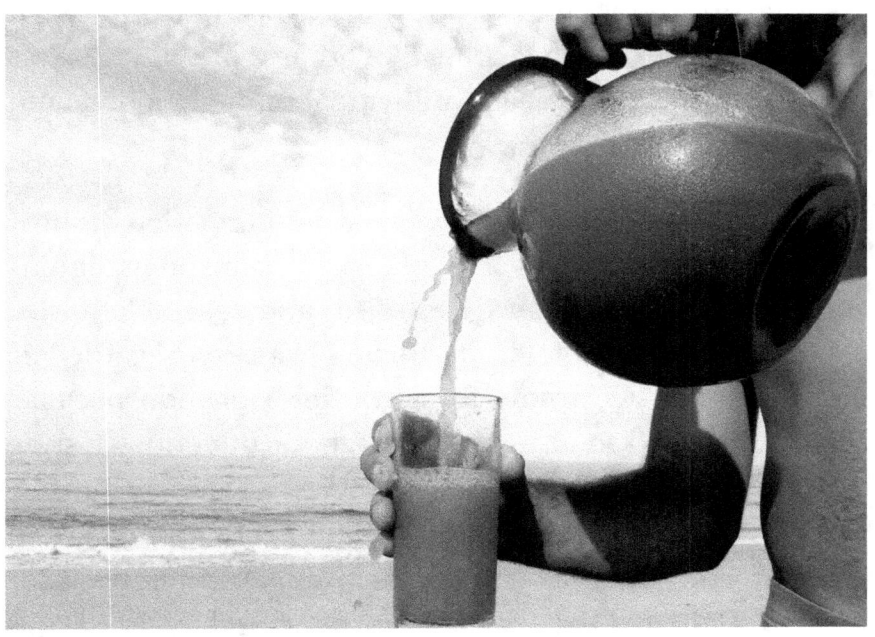

Toxins routinely enter our bodies easily from a variety of sources. This can be due to the foods we eat, drinks we consume, and even from the air we breathe. As we consume more and more food and drinks that have been processed and contain preservatives, many have been treated with chemicals that are not healthy for our body. The body normally works to get rid of these toxins; however, it cannot simply eliminate all of the toxins that have accumulated from years of living with unhealthy practices. Some individuals who have increased levels of toxins in their bodies begin to experience ill effects, often requiring medication.

To help our bodies get rid of toxins, one of the best options can be a juice fast. Juice fasting is considered an effective and safe method for detoxifying our bodies with the help of fruits, vegetables and water. Unlike other kinds of fasting, juice fasting provides the body with the nourishment it needs. However, juice fasting, like other types of fasts, has different aspects that each individual should understand before committing to one.

As a type of detox diet that involves a certain period of time, a juice fast is where an individual only consumes liquids such as water, herbal teas, fresh fruit and vegetable juices, and strained vegetable broth. Juicing has been regarded as one of the most extreme forms of detoxification because there is no solid food intake throughout the entire fasting process. As much as possible, when juice fasting occurs, it is advised that you not take in any liquids that put a strain on your body such as soda, coffee, milk, protein powder mixes, caffeinated teas, pasteurized juice, and the like.

When I first learned of some of these guidelines, I remember thinking that I really did not have too much trouble in this area of liquids that strain my body. However, there was NO way I was going to give up coffee during a fast. I've eliminated coffee from my diet on many different occasions—pregnancy being the biggest, and only because I was quite nauseated—but I always go back to drinking it. I have even given up drinking coffee for several weeks at different times in my life, just to prove to myself that I could do it.

All to say, going into my first juice fast, I made a decision I was not going to quit drinking coffee throughout the day because I knew I would go right back to it. You may disagree with this and that is just fine with me. Like I said in the introduction, a juice fast is a personal journey.

People decide to juice fast for a variety of reasons and utilize different methods. Advocates of juicing claim they experience rejuvenating effects like healing from medical conditions like skin infections, kidney disorders, arthritis, high blood pressure and others. Healing can occur because juice fasting helps to eliminate toxins while increasing nutrients in the body that are necessary to energize its natural regenerative abilities.

Individuals who decide to pursue juice fasting should prepare for it, as the preparation process can sometimes determine how well, or how poorly your fast will turn out. Making plans ahead of time (supplies and food needed) can lead to a successful and rewarding juice fast.

According to proponents of juice fasting, many prefer to conduct one during the warmer months of the year, spring being one of the most suitable.[2] Personally, I've now done it at least once during each of the four seasons and I would have to say that summer is probably my favorite because of all the fresh fruits and vegetables available for juicing.

At the same time, you should also decide on how many days you want to fast. For those who prefer to fast for only one to three days, doing it over the space of a weekend is recommended. Try to free up your weekend from any appointments or errands you usually do, especially if this will be your first time. Since you don't know what to expect, you will want to stay close to home.

When I first start a juice fast, the first day is rather uneventful. However, during the second day, my body does a major "clean out" so I do not want to be too far from my own bathroom. Enough said!

Once you have made your decisions, you will want to visit your local grocery store and purchase a wide variety of fresh fruits and vegetables. If you have never juiced before, it will be difficult for you to know how much to purchase until you begin to see how much juice you get from different fruits and vegetables.

The first time I ever juiced, I was amazed at how much juice you can get from a head of romaine lettuce, and how little kale and spinach make. It will simply take some experimentation on your part to discover what fruits and vegetables you like in your juices and how much the different fruits and vegetables will produce.

One of the recommendations I read suggested that at least seven days prior to fasting, begin cutting down or eliminating intake of the following: alcohol, caffeine, cigarettes, drugs, over-the-counter medicines, sugar, salt, artificial sweeteners, meat, fried foods, microwaved or processed foods, dairy products, and gluten-rich foods like oats, barley, rye, wheat bread, pasta, pies, cakes and pastries. At the same time, try to increase your intake of raw foods in your diet such as salads and sprouted foods, pure water and hydrating fluids, herbal teas, fresh fruit and vegetable juices, plus leafy green vegetables and vegetable soups.

While I did many of these things, I didn't do them all. Like I said, I continued to drink my coffee with Half and Half, but I did cut back on pastas and grains.

Certain individuals should be careful before deciding to juice fast. It is best to speak with your doctor, especially if you are malnourished and underweight, a lactating mother, or diagnosed with cancer or ulcers. Additionally, individuals with poor or low immune systems or post-operative patients should check with their medical practitioner before attempting a juice fast.

In order to be successful in your juice fast, you should have both discipline and determination leading up to your fast, during the fast, and after this process is over. If you are a "starter" and not a "finisher," you may want to pick a short period of time to do your first juice fast. You want to feel successful when you do this. If you suspect you will have trouble seeing this through, go easy on yourself. Pick a weekend. You will learn a lot in just a couple of days which will help prepare you for future ventures.

What Are the Nutritional Benefits of Juicing Produce?

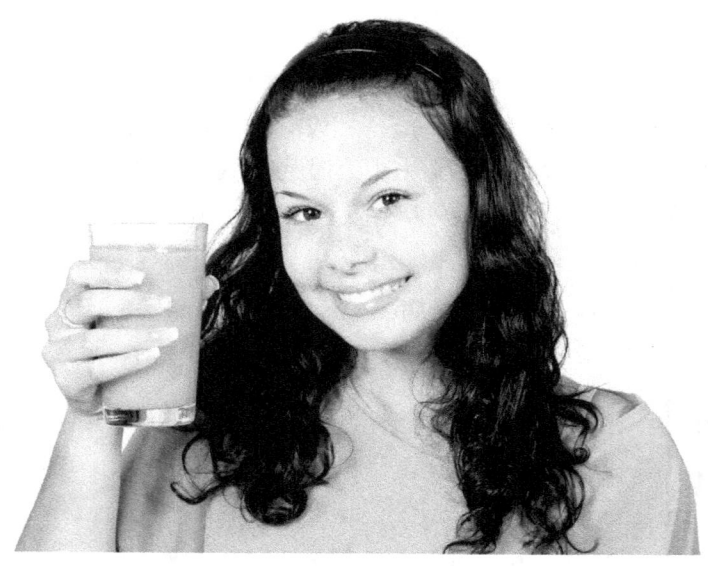

Fasting has many proven benefits, making it a popular method for individuals who want to detoxify their bodies. When choosing a juice fast, the most preferred ingredients are organic fruits and vegetables. Organic is preferable because one of the main objectives of this particular method is to rid your body of toxins.

Although it may be difficult for you to afford organic produce, try to buy the best quality you can afford. Additionally, there are some products that are "sturdier" than others. For instance, try to buy organic strawberries and other berries because their skins are so thin and fragile.

However, fruits such as oranges, pineapples, and cucumbers are ones where you will eliminate their peelings before juicing.

In an effort to help you understand the nutritional benefits of juicing, I have included some information below.

High nutritional content. As you may know, juice is a natural source of water that is rich in proteins, carbohydrates, vitamins, and minerals. At the same time, juice is also abundant in essential fatty acids, enzymes, carotenes, chlorophyll, and flavonoids. When found in juices, these nutrients are in a form that our bodies can quickly absorb.

Most of the nutrition you get from juice is not usually found in foods we consume whole because cooking food can cause some nutrients to be lost during cooking. For instance, vitamins A, D, E, and K are water-soluble vitamins that are susceptible to heat. Juicing helps preserve these vitamins and minerals because they are not heated. This results in sustained or increased nutrition for your body.

Juice fasting provides your body with efficient, high-quality nutrition. Additional nutrition is possible with juicing since the juicer already does most of the work your body would do in separating nutrients. As a result, you can experience a quick increase in energy that is helpful when performing certain physical activities that burn more calories or fats because your body does not have to work so hard.

Enhances digestion. As I just stated, juicing means your body does not need to work as hard to break it food. Supporters of juicing claim it helps make the digestive process easier on the body, while vitamins and minerals enter the system faster than usual.

Helps clean the liver. Liver detoxification is one of the benefits of juicing. Detoxification occurs because of the high amount of antioxidants, vitamins and other nutrients acquired from juicing that assist your liver in ridding itself of toxins and waste, resulting in a cleaner, healthier and well-functioning liver.[3]

Aids you in losing weight. Both fruits and vegetables are helpful for weight loss so an increase in fruit and vegetable consumption through juicing has the potential to enhance weight loss effects. My initial motivation for juicing was a desire to lose weight, which I did. In addition, consuming juices have been shown to improve both blood sugar and blood pressure levels when your diet is restricted to just juicing.[4]

Emotional and physical enhancement. When the internal parts of your body achieve balance through juice fasting, emotional and physical attachment to food tends to diminish, helping individuals achieve greater overall health and wellbeing.[5] When I did an extended juice fast of 30 days, I found that my cravings for sugar almost disappeared. That was huge for me and continues to be true to this day.

The benefits mentioned above are just a few of the ones juicing can provide. Juicing is not only for individuals who are experiencing certain medical conditions, but also for those who wish to maintain a healthy lifestyle. Once you check with your doctor (especially if you have an underlying medical condition), you can begin your juice fasting experience.

Juicing really helped to break through my love for sugar and candy. Choosing to only drink juices for a long juice fast helped me appreciate the sweetness of fruits that I did not have before.

Is Juicing Really As Healthy As It Claims to Be?

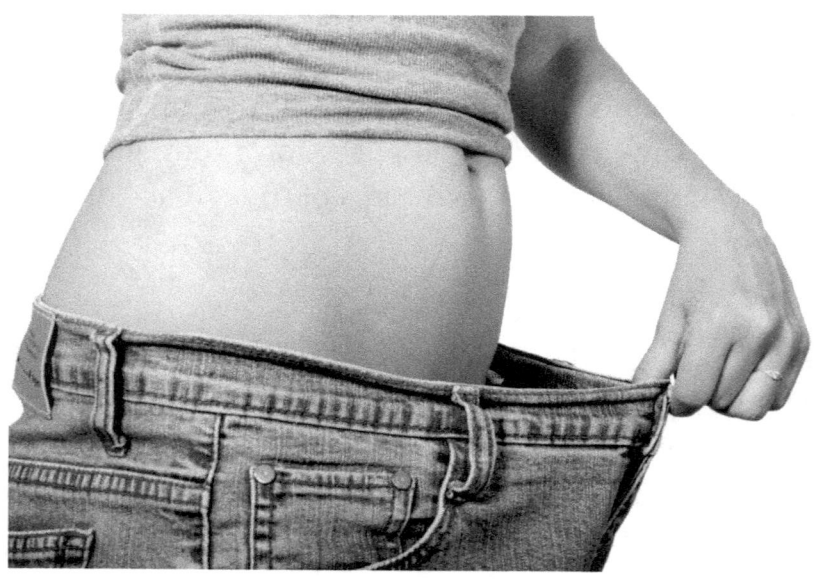

Put simply, juicing is the process of extracting juices from raw fruits and vegetables using a juice extractor. Extractors grind and spin down the fruits and vegetables, separating the juice from its pulp.

One of the well-known philosophies of juice fasting is that the juice extracted from raw fruits and vegetables has special enzymes that promote health of your digestive system.[6] At the same time, supporters of juice fasting claim that it can help boost the immune system, aiding the fight against negative health conditions such as cancer or kidney problems.[7]

Juicing is said to have the ability to correct imbalances in the body while boosting energy to perform physical activities. Other individuals state that juicing fights aging and rids the body of toxins.[8] What is the real science behind juicing? Is it as healthy as others claim it to be?

According to Debra J. Johnston, RD, Director of Nutrition Services at Remuda Ranch, "Juicing may be a good way for individuals who do not consume enough fruits and vegetables to get important vitamins and minerals by creating tasty concoctions of fruit and vegetable juice."[9] However, she adds that the juicing process may eliminate the fiber found in fruits and vegetables, which is necessary for healthy digestion.[10]

Jennifer K. Nelson, a nutritionist from the Mayo Clinic, supports Johnston's statement, "Juicing probably is not any healthier than eating whole fruits and vegetables. Juicing extracts the juice from fresh fruits or vegetables. The resulting liquid contains most of the vitamins, minerals and plant chemicals (phytonutrients) found in the whole fruit. However, whole fruits and vegetables also have healthy fiber, which is lost during most juicing."[11]

Fiber is found in most fruits and vegetables, and is fundamental in the prevention of certain health issues: 1) diabetes mellitus is prevented through the maintenance of blood sugar levels, 2) cardiovascular diseases are hindered by getting rid of excessive cholesterol in the body through the digestive tract, and 3) obesity is halted by providing the sensation of fullness in between meals.[12]

Furthermore, juicing can also increase caloric intake; most freshly squeezed fruit juices are actually calorie dense, especially pineapple and banana juices. (Seldom will you ever extract juice from a banana in a juicer because it is too mushy). When an individual consumes a lot of fruit juice, the carbohydrate load may increase, causing a rapid surge in blood sugar levels. Obese individuals with high blood pressure, diabetes or high cholesterol must first consult with their physicians before attempting a juice fast because this may exacerbate their present medical condition.[13] Definitely some good advice.

The bottom line is: juicing certainly has its health benefits but precautions must be taken before considering this kind of fasting. Especially for those who suffer from underlying medical conditions, it is best to consult with an attending physician before beginning a juice fast. First timers should also discuss this type of diet change with experts so they know how to properly perform juice fasting and to experience as few negative side effects as possible.

Are There Any Negatives to Juicing?

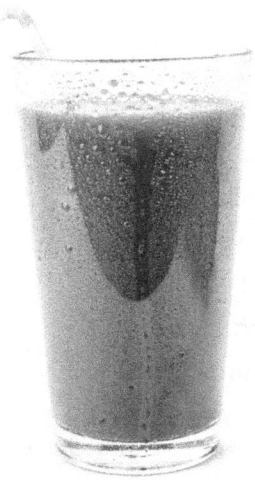

Juicing has been enjoying popularity these days as its proponents claim that juicing produces numerous health benefits. Some include better absorption of nutrients, prevention of certain illnesses, and enhanced digestion. However, there are some disadvantages to be aware of before committing to juice fasting.

Loss of Fiber. A surprising fact about juicing is that it actually sacrifices fiber. When fruits or vegetables are juiced, the water and nutrients from the pulp are discarded. (You can freeze the pulp to be used later if you wish). If you do not plan to add the excess pulp to your soups or other foods, you are throwing away fiber that is important for proper digestion, the absorption of nutrients, the maintenance of colon health, lowering of cholesterol and an aid for the prevention of constipation.

High glycemic index. Fruits usually have a higher glycemic index than vegetables, meaning different foods cause various spikes of the blood sugar levels in your body. The juice in some fruits and vegetables will usually contain higher sugar levels than their whole fruits or vegetables because there is a higher concentration. This is not a great situation, especially for individuals diagnosed with diabetes mellitus, obesity or any cardiovascular conditions.[14]

Long preparation time. Although juicing can be quicker to prepare than cooking a meal, it can certainly take some time to peel and cut fruits and vegetables. For busy individuals like students, working parents, or moms looking after their children, juicing can be labor intensive. Realistically, cleaning, chopping, extracting and cleanup after you have finished making your juice may consume more time and effort than simply eating the fruit or vegetable itself.

When I would make fruit and vegetable juices, I would make enough to produce about one gallon of each. This usually meant it took me about two hours to make enough juice to last me three to four days at a time. Since I do not enjoy cleaning my juicer, I made enough and stored it in glass canning jars with plastic lids. Although my juice may not have been fresh right when I drank it, the time I saved over the course of several days by not having to clean my juicer several times a day was worth it to me.

Time consuming disinfecting and cleaning. Fresh juices are consumed raw; therefore, after each use of the juicing equipment, you will need to thoroughly clean it. This includes the juicer itself, its parts, the cutting board, knives, storage containers, and other utensils. Although dishwashers can clean some materials, other utensils need a thorough washing by hand. This is another reason why I made my juice in big batches so that clean up only had to happen every few days.

Juice fasting is expensive. Juice fasting requires a juicer, high quality knives, storage containers, and for the best results, organic fruits and vegetables. (As I mentioned earlier, do the best you can afford). The cost of the juicer depends upon the type, brand and model you choose. Juicers typically range from $200 to $300 so the expense of juicing requires some monetary investment.

Raw fruits and vegetables contain microbes. Certain microbes such as E. coli and salmonella are actually found in raw vegetables and fruits and can cause gastroenteritis, food poisoning, or can even be fatal. Some of these microbes can only be removed through heat, which are negated when juicing. This is why individuals with cancer or poor immune systems should reconsider before trying a juice fast.

Is Juicing Just As Good As Eating Whole Fruits & Vegetables?

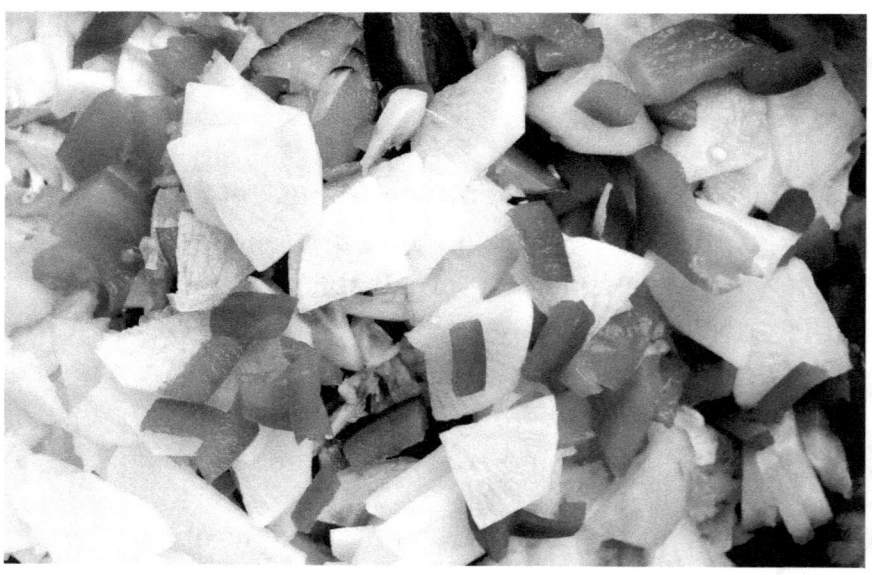

Juicing is certainly a great way to introduce or add more fruits and vegetables into your regular diet. For me, I had never purchased kale until I read that it was nutritious in juice. Although drinking juice offers a great deal of health benefits, it has never been proven that juicing is better than eating the actual vegetable or fruit itself. However, nowadays, experts are recommending a combination of both.[15]

Juicing is different from eating whole fruits and vegetables because the extracted juice contains all the vitamins, minerals and other nutrients that are part of the produce.

However, juicing leaves behind the fiber that is also necessary for our health, especially when it comes to our digestive system. This is one reason why juicing cannot replace eating the actual fruit or vegetable whole.

Because juicing eliminates the fiber found in fruits and vegetables, the juice is absorbed by our bodies much more rapidly than in its solid form. The digestive system needs to work less to properly digest the nutrients, making the nourishment found in these foods available almost instantly for the body to use. Since the nutrient absorption is immediate, a person can quickly feel an increase in physical energy.

Juicing can provide an ideal way for individuals who are not into eating vegetables to obtain the nutrients and vitamins they provide. For instance; if you are having trouble with adding more vegetables to your diet, you can actually consume more just by juicing them.

If you dislike the taste of vegetables such as spinach, broccoli or kale, you can juice them and combine the juice of these greens with the juice of apples, pineapples, mangoes, and other fruits. The sweetness from the fruit juice will dominate the drink's taste so it can make it easier for you to consume the drink.

Eating fruits and vegetables is certainly healthy. Based on a 1997 report published by the World Cancer Research Fund on the Vegetarianism and Vegan Nutrition website, a predominantly plant-based diet regimen that is loaded with fruits and vegetables can actually lower the risk of cancer.[16]

However, if you do not enjoy eating fruits and vegetables, especially when they are raw, juicing can provide a way for you to still get the nutrients your body needs. The University of California, Davis conducted a study on juicing and cancer, and showed that individuals who consume vegetable juices together with eating whole vegetables are more likely to consume the recommended daily amount.[17]

While fiber is an important element in our diets, juicing is something no one does indefinitely. Except in severe medical cases, people are going to return to solid foods meaning fiber will eventually return to their diet as they resume eating the actual fruits and vegetables.

Is Fresh Juice Better Than Commercially Processed Juice?

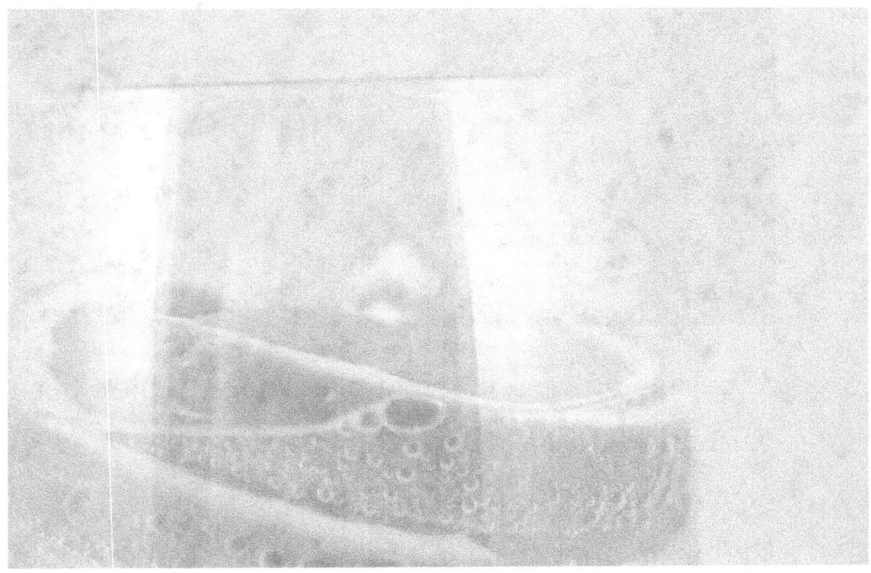

Are you wondering whether those commercially processed juices you are seeing popping up in the health food stores and supermarkets are healthier than fresh juices? Well, you are not alone. Most people actually think that drinking processed juice, especially ones labeled natural or organic, have the same healthy ingredients, compounds and nutrients as those freshly made by you. There are several important differences between processed, canned or bottled juices compared to juice freshly made. Below are some distinct differences between the two:

Processed or Canned Juices

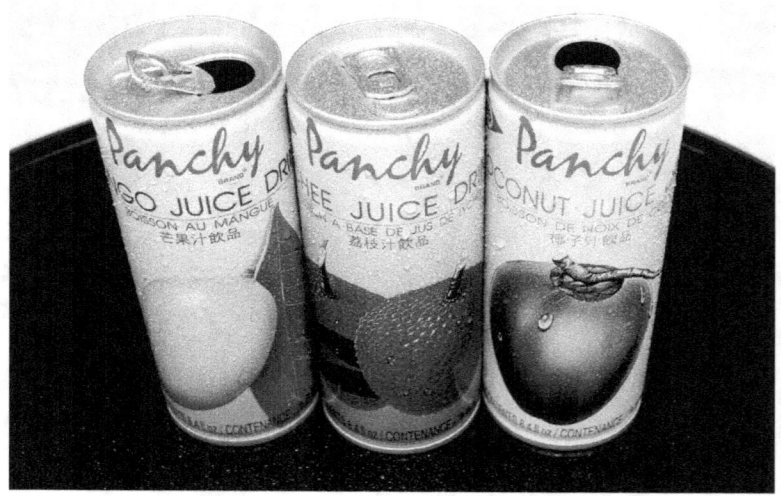

–   Almost all processed or commercial juices have been pasteurized. This means they have been heated to high temperatures. This can actually destroy vitamins, minerals and other nutrients found in fruits and vegetables. Furthermore, it can alter the flavor and smell of the juice itself.[18]

–   Manufacturers and processors of commercial juices will often add chemical or manufactured "flavor packs" to replace the fruit flavors and aromas lost during the heating process. These chemicals come from orange-derived substances, oils, and essences that improve the overall flavor of juice.[19] However, some researchers have shown that this particular addition has been the cause behind certain allergic reactions of individuals drinking processed juices.

– Most processed juices are fruit concentrates and are not 100% juice. In fact, they do not contain the whole fruit or vegetable because they are largely made from water as well as sugar. This is not healthy—especially for individuals with diabetes, obesity, or cardiovascular conditions.[20]

– Since most commercial juices are placed in bottles or cans, metal, wax and other chemicals in the containers can mix with the juice.[21]

– Some imported juices may have traces of banned pesticides.[22]

– Every gram of carbohydrates indicated in the packaging of the juice comes directly from sugar.

– Even though the *sugar* in processed juice is derived naturally from the fruit, when the juice is processed, all its natural fibers, vitamins and minerals can be lost.

Freshly Made Juices

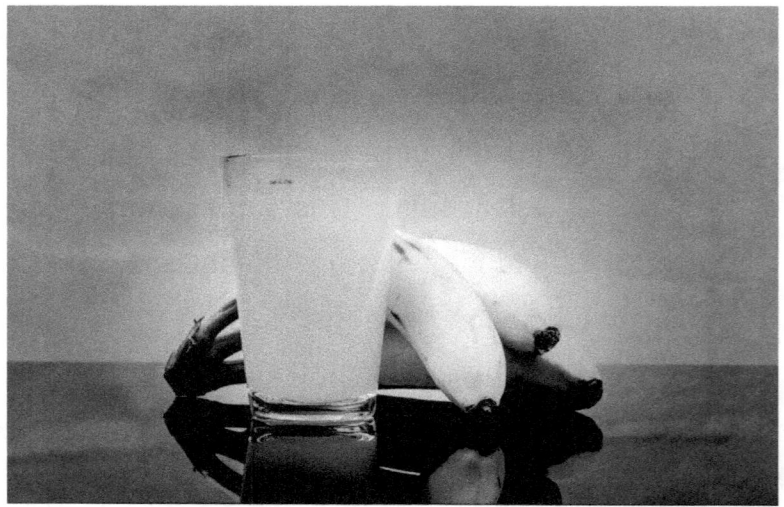

- Unlike processed or commercial juices, freshly extracted juices do not go through heat or pasteurization. Because of this, they maintain all of the original vitamins, minerals, fluids, enzymes, amino acids, chlorophyll and other nutrients of the fruit or vegetable.

- Because it's naturally extracted, freshly made juice helps the body in different ways – by promoting growth and development, easing the digestive processes, increasing energy, renewing and protecting cells from oxidation and free radical damage, and purifying and enriching the blood.[23]

– A great and healthy alternative for kids who are not inclined to eating fruits and vegetables

If you want to achieve the most benefits from drinking fruit and vegetable juices, it is best to learn how to extract fresh juice the right way. Do not settle for pasteurized processed juices as they do not contain the nutrients you need and could even lead to health problems.

It is simple to make freshly extracted juices with the help of a good juicer. Just remember, it takes time to prepare many of the fruits and vegetables you will use, and cleaning up the machines and utensils used can be lengthy.

You can find many juice recipes online that will instruct you step-by-step and show you ways to add spice to your juices' overall taste and flavor.

How Long Should I Stay on a Juice Fast?

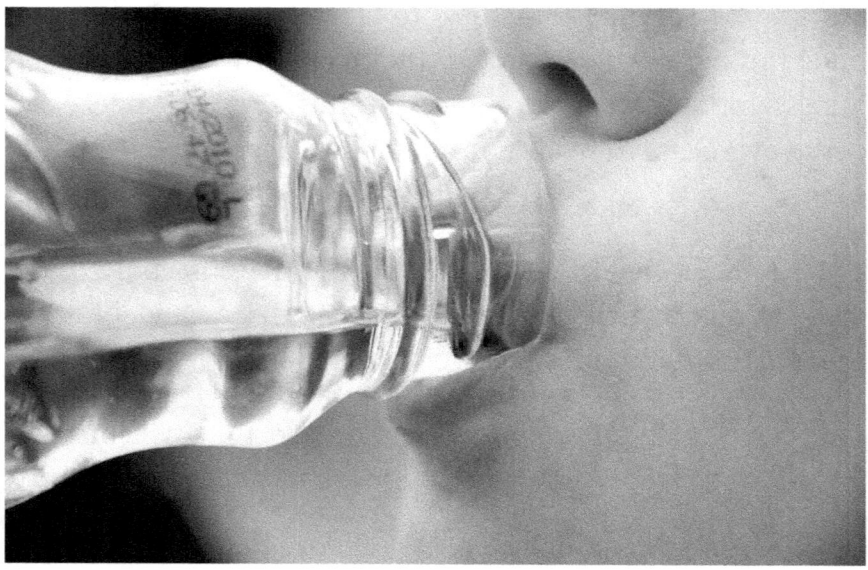

People diet or fast for different reasons. Most individuals fast as a means to lose weight, others desire spiritual refreshment, while some simply want to cleanse their bodies of toxins. These are also some of the same reasons that determine the length of fasting. Everyone is different, and our bodies work differently as well. The length of a juice fast can vary widely from one to sixty days.

Personally, I have conducted several juice fasts. My first one lasted 13 days. Then I took two days off because of social commitments I had made previously, then I returned to juice fasting for another 13 days. Another time I fasted for 30 days; and still another was only 10 days.

You might be wondering: How long should I stay on a juice fast? What is the ideal length of time? Is shorter or longer better?

A long juice fast is more preferable to a short one. However, if it is your first time fasting, it is best to start with a fast that lasts one to five days so that you and your body can adjust to the entire process. As with so many health situations, it is important to listen to your body and know your limitations. Because I am in excellent health, my first attempts at juice fasting were longer than this. However, I also gave myself permission to quit at any time I felt my health might suffer.

It is important to get your doctor's permission to juice fast as juice fasting is not for everyone. Although it is recommended and safe for most individuals, juice fasting is not safe for individuals with medical conditions such as diabetes, gout, metabolic syndrome, pregnancy or during lactation. If you are not sure, always consult with your physician regarding this matter.

Once you have determined whether you are qualified to juice fast, you can start with one day and then fast for two days—slowly increasing up to five days. For beginners who desire to do a five-day juice fast, it is best to begin fasting during the weekend. This will give you time at home and a flexible schedule as you begin to understand and see how fasting will affect your body.

Remember to listen to your body. Even if your mind wants to meet the predetermined number of days of fasting but your body is not cooperating, do not push it. Always stop if you are encountering problems and listen to your body so you will know if you can carry on with fasting.

During one particular fast, I had gone for two weeks. My plan was to go longer, but sometime during the day, I just felt as though I really needed to eat food instead of drink it, so that is exactly what I did. Instead of continuing, I gave myself permission to end the fast and return to eating whole foods.

When you achieve an effortless five-day juice fast, you can try to stretch the length of fasting further—to seven or ten days, until you reach thirty or even forty days. Longer juice fasting is actually possible, especially if you are used to fasting and you have already mastered some of the problems you might encounter during the first few days, such as how to handle hunger pangs.

Prolonged fasting can actually be beneficial to the body as it undergoes an uninterrupted time of repair, cleansing and healing. At the same time, most individuals who have tried prolonged fasting—approximately 30 to 40 days—have experienced several changes in their body. These changes can include increased and improved mental clarity, enhanced emotional, physical and spiritual sensitivity, healthy weight loss, increased energy levels, a better complexion, reduced water retention, and other benefits.

Personally, after I had been on a 30-day fast, I found that I slept better and was not hungry in between times as I thought I would be. My usual regiment when I juice is to have 16 ounces of fresh fruit juice in the morning, following by two to three more 16 ounce servings of vegetable juice throughout the day.

As with any change in your diet, consult the information I have presented so far so that you can make an educated decision of when you will fast, how long you will fast, and what juices you will make when you fast.

How Do I Break a Juice Fast?

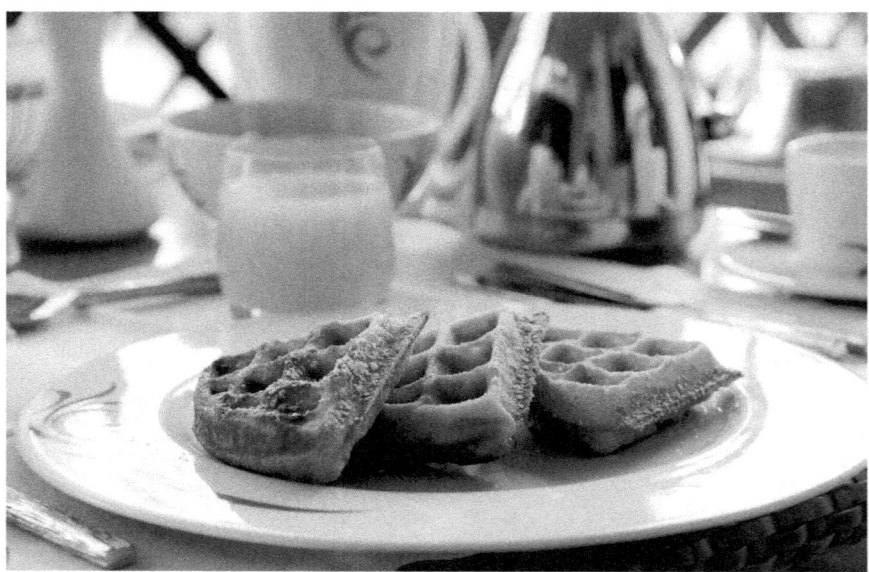

Juice fasting offers many health benefits, specifically the chance for the body to rest from digestive processes. Juicing allows the body's energy to focus on cleansing itself through eliminating toxins, waste and dead cells. The vitamins, minerals and other nutrients the body receives from juice fasting are utilized in repairing, cleansing, toning and healing the entire body.

When quitting or breaking a juice fast, you should do it in a way that your body will continue to eliminate toxins. This can be achieved by slowly breaking the fasting process as you allow the body to switch from cleansing mode back to its regular digestive mode.

It is important to follow your instincts since your body knows best. It will let you know whether you are breaking the fast the right way or not. Furthermore, do not be tempted to consume foods and drinks you had been craving during your fast. Doing so can actually cause some digestive issues as your stomach has become accustomed to only consuming fruit and vegetable juices for quite some time.

If you have done a prolonged juice fast, take more precautions and reintroduce food into your body in a much slower manner, as well as in small amounts. It is advised that you keep your meals very light or even raw during the first few days of breaking your fast.

Avoid greasy foods and foods rich in fats, starch, processed sugar and salt, as these can cause headaches and nausea. Instead, choose whole fresh fruits and steamed vegetables. It is also a good idea to chew your food well as the enzymes found in your saliva will help in the digestive process. In turn, this will offer less stress to your digestive system while it is still returning to its usual mode.

Another great way to properly break a juice fast includes consuming fruit and vegetable juices while slowly adding whole raw fruits and vegetables with high water content—such as grapes and tomatoes—into your diet. You can also include raw light salads with dressing, or perhaps light vegetable soups as your meals. Increase the amount of food slowly over the next two to three days.

A sample menu for breaking a juice fast is based on *The Juice Lady's Guide to Juicing for Health* by Cherie Calbom. Her advice includes the following: For breakfast, you can have fresh juice or a smoothie, a slice of fruit or a vegetable salad plus herbal tea; for your morning snacks, you can take any fresh juice; for lunch, raw soup or a lightly cooked vegetable soup with a salad; for your afternoon snacks, any fresh juice; for dinner, lightly steamed vegetables, vegetable soup and salad; and for your evening snack, fresh vegetable juice or an herbal tea. [24]

By keeping these things in mind, you can help your body achieve a smooth transition from fruit and vegetable juices to lightly cooked vegetables and soups as you return to your usual healthy diet in a proper and safe way.

How Do I Choose a Juicer?

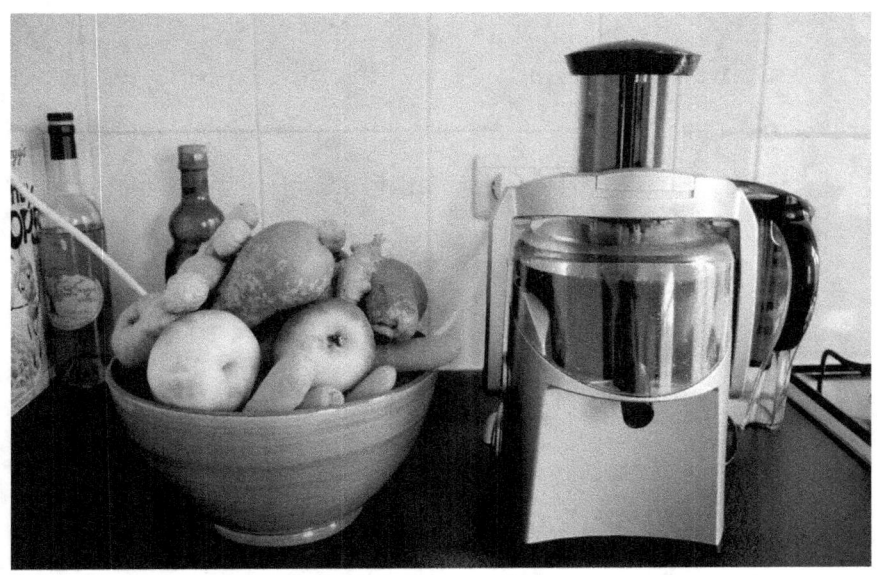

Juicing fresh fruits and vegetables at home offers many health benefits. These drinks provide the body with bioflavonoids, enzymes, vitamins, minerals, antioxidants and other nutrients necessary to keep our bodies healthy and strong. However, to make this possible and easier for you, you should have your own juicer. Having your own appliance is an excellent alternative to buying expensive juice drinks in the grocery store that often contain high amounts of sugar and preservatives.

Having your own juicer allows you to make your own beverages, letting you customize the flavor combinations perfect for you and your family. Below is a guide to help you choose the right juicer that will meet your needs and fit your budget.

Type of Juicers. At present, the market has six different kinds of juicers. They are as follows:

- **Centrifugal** – Considered the most affordable type, centrifugal juicers are also the most popular choice. They are perfect for individuals with a limited budget. The centrifugal juicer comes with a disc that spins the juice out, catching the remaining pulp in the basket.

- **Citrus** – Sold both as a manual and an electric model, this type is perfect for juicing citrus fruits.

- **Manual** – With these you will need to use your own muscles to squeeze out the juice on your own using a cheesecloth to filter out the pulp.

- **Masticating** – Known for producing juice that does not have any foam. This type is perfect for baby sauces, baby food, and sorbets. You will be using a fine screen in producing the juice.

- **Triturating** – This type makes use of twin gears to shred, and then press the juice out from the fruits and vegetables. Although more expensive than the other selections, triturating juicers extract more juice.

- **Wheatgrass** – Able to juice wheatgrass—a unique feature that you cannot get with other types of juicers.

Power and size. The greater the power of the juicer, the better. You will not need to chop fruits or vegetables extensively when you buy a juicer with a powerful motor. In addition, juicing with a more powerful juicer is often quicker. For homes with small kitchen counters or cabinet space, size will be another thing to consider when shopping for a juicer.

Ease of use. If you prefer a juicer that is easy to use and clean, then choose a simple one. However, if you are not in a hurry and you want to spend a little more time juicing, then you can purchase a more complex type, especially if it has additional features that you think you can use.

Budget. Set aside a specific amount you want to spend for your juicer. A basic juicer can cost around $30 while high-quality designs and well-known brands can cost up to $300.

Longevity. This is specifically important to individuals who purchase the more expensive juicers. This equipment is surely an investment, so it is a good idea to make sure that it can last a long time—especially its motors—and make sure it has a warranty from the manufacturer. Typically, the higher quality brands of juicers offer great customer service, affordable repair and return policies in case you experience problems over time.

Personally, I purchased a Breville Juice Fountain® Duo. We found a refurbished one with the warranties and have thoroughly enjoyed it. It is one of the more expensive models out there, but it works beautifully and allows me to put in whole apples, grapes with the stems on them, and other "shortcuts." The Breville website offers all the parts for sale so if I ever need to replace any of the parts, I can buy them easily online.

What Are Some Recipes I Could Make to Get Started?

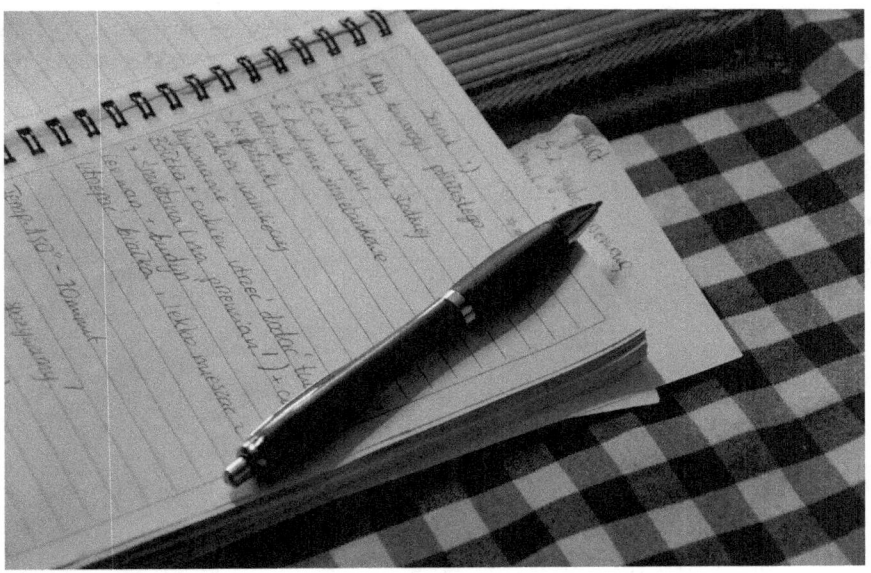

Juicing actually does not need recipes. You can simply extract the juice from your favorite fruits or vegetables and try different combinations each time. You can combine the juice of fruits and vegetables together to create healthy and delicious drinks. It is advisable to do this because most vegetable juices produce a bitter taste while most fruit juices are too sweet and acidic and can cause stomach upset. To avoid the possibility of negative side effects, it is advised you use both vegetables and fruits in making your juices.

When I am juicing, my fruit juices are almost always different. Depending upon what we have available in the house that needs juiced (because nobody wants to eat them—mushy grapes, strawberries, and apples) and what I buy at the store, I have created some incredible fruit juices. No recipes—just juiced whatever I felt like.

With vegetable juices, I have a little bit more structure to my recipes. Here is my basic green juice. (Remember, I make a big batch when I do this so if you want something smaller in quantity, you will have to reduce the amounts).

Jennifer's Green Juice

- 2 - 4 cups coconut water
- 2 big heads of romaine lettuce
- 2 bunches of fresh spinach
- 4 large kale leaves
- 10 large carrots
- 2 large cucumbers, peeled
- 4 tomatoes
- 2 limes, peeled
- 6 apples
- 3 pears
- 1 to 2 inch piece of fresh ginger, peeled

Then, I process everything through the juicer. When I pour myself a drink, I like to add salt and pepper to it while enjoying it over ice.

Sometimes I have put in some yellow squash, zucchini, bell peppers and beets. I did not care very much for the time when I added cabbage, onion or garlic. Just experiment once you feel comfortable and find a basic recipe you like.

Below are some other good tasting juice recipes you can start with as you begin your journey into juice fasting.

Salsa Verde with a Kick

Ingredients:

- 2 bell peppers, seeded and core removed
- 1 bunch of green onions (the whole thing)
- 1 bunch fresh cilantro
- 3 large tomatoes
- ½-inch slice Jalapeno pepper
- ½ avocado
- 1 teaspoon taco seasoning
- Juice from 1 lime

Directions:

1. Using your juicer, process the peppers, cilantro, green onions, Jalapeno pepper and tomatoes

2. Place the avocado into a blender

3. Add a little bit of the fresh juice you just made to the blender

4. Process until the avocado is finely chopped

5. Now add the rest of the fresh juice

6. Add the taco seasoning and lime juice

Delightful Squash

Ingredients:

- 2 yellow squash
- 3 carrots
- 3 cups fresh pumpkin, diced
- 2 cups butternut squash, diced

Directions:

1. Wash the squash and carrots

2. Cut off any stems

3. Take the seeds out of the pumpkin and squash and remove the peeling of the pumpkin and squash

4. Process the ingredients in your juicer

5. Pour into a container and shake before pouring

Watermelon Juice with Protein

Ingredients:

- 4 cups fresh watermelon
- 2 cups fresh blackberries or blueberries
- 1 heaping scoop of your favorite protein powder

Directions:

1. Remove the watermelon from the rind and measure
2. Wash the berries
3. Process the watermelon and berries through the juicer
4. Pour into a glass and stir in the protein powder

Spicy Cucumber

Ingredients:

- 1 lime, peeled
- 2 bunches fresh cilantro
- 2 apples
- 3 cucumbers, peeled
- Little dash of hot sauce

Directions:

1. Process the lime, cilantro, apples, and cucumbers through the juicer
2. Pour the juice into a glass or drinking container
3. Add a few dashes of hot sauce and stir it in
4. Add ice if desired and enjoy

Blue Protein Power

Ingredients:

- 2 cups fresh blueberries
- 2 cups fresh red grapes
- 2 large kale leaves
- 1 scoop of your favorite protein powder

Directions:

1. Rinse the blueberries, grapes, and kale leaves
2. Process these through your juicer
3. Pour the juice into a drinking container
4. Stir in the protein powder
5. Add ice if desired

Conclusion

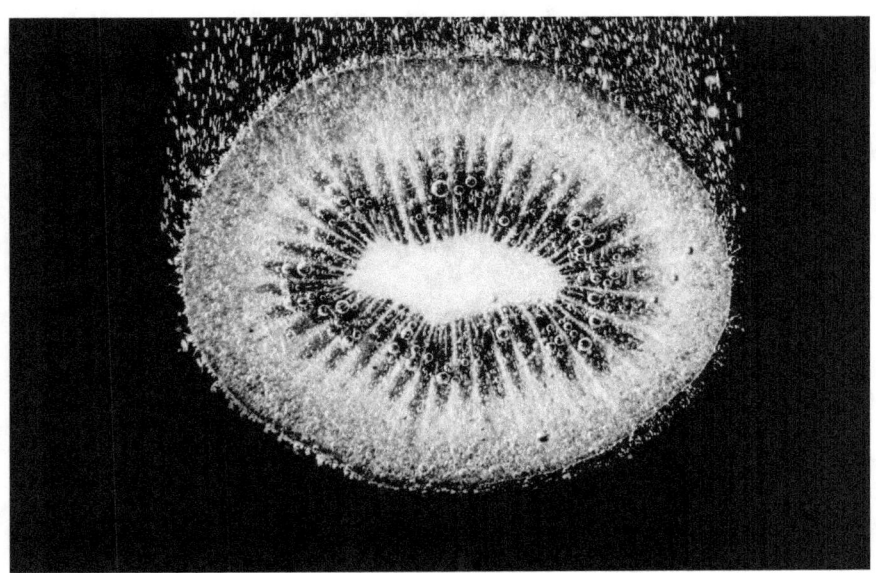

Welcome to the end of the book!

Now that you have finished the book, I want to thank you for your purchase and I would greatly appreciate it if you would go over to Amazon where you bought your copy and leave a review.

http://www.amazon.com/Juice-Health-Benefits-Wellness-ebook/dp/B009NOSZSS/

Your thoughts and comments will help to make my next resource better.

Thank you!

Acknowledgements

Many thanks to the following photographers from Flickr.com for the use or their artwork in this book.

- corbin_dana
- mathiasbaert
- raleighwoman
- Florena_Presse
- Diekatrin
- Stiftelsen Elektronikkbransjen
- Kirti Poddar
- Patrick Hoesly

Additional Resources

Additional works by Jennifer Wells:

Going Gluten Free:
A Quick Start Guide for a Gluten-Free Diet

Top 10 Tips to Help You Lose Weight

About the Author

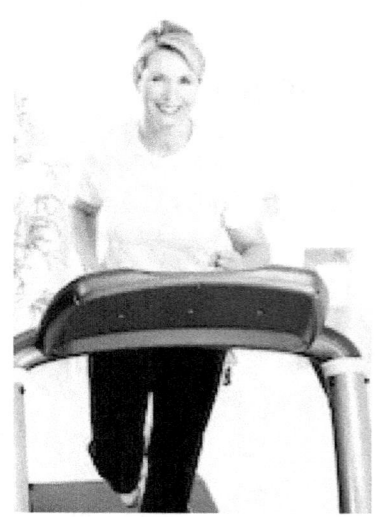

Always into sports and very active growing up, Jennifer never gave much thought to diet and exercise. Weight gain was not much of an issue. Then, after marriage and the birth of her twin boys, Jennifer noticed she had problems keeping her weight under control.

After numerous years of frustration, trying to get rid of stubborn pounds and not feeling as well as she wanted, Jennifer began her own personal research into diet and exercise. As a result, she ended up going back to school to get a degree in nutritional science.

Now she enjoys living a healthy lifestyle, spending time outdoors, teaching classes on nutrition at her local high school, and sharing healthy tips and information with family and friends.

And just in case you were curious, Jennifer is now back down to her weight before she had her four children.

Endnotes

[1] "History of Juicing." Viewed online at http://www.earthturns.com/History-Juicing-a/152.htm on 10.02.12.

[2] "Juice Fasting." Viewed online at http://www.jeffreywarber.com/hc%20pages/juicefasting.html on 10.01.12.

[3] Lyn Vaccaro, "Raw Juice: A Natural Liver Cleanse to Restore Healthy Liver Function," November 12, 2008. Viewed online at http://voices.yahoo.com/raw-juice-natural-liver-cleanse-restore-healthy-2144854.html on 10.01.12.

[4] Healthy-Vegetable-Gardening.com, "Juicing for Diabetics Juice that Works!" Viewed online at http://www.healthy-vegetable-gardening.com/juicingfordiabetics.html on 10.02.12.

[5] "Spiritual Organic Juice Fasting." Viewed online at http://treeoflife.nu on 10.02.12.

[6] Chris Iliades, MD, "Is Juicing Good for Digestive Health?" Viewed online at http://www.everydayhealth.com/digestive-health/is-juicing-good-for-digestive-health.aspx on 10.02.12.

[7] Ibid.

[8] Ibid.

[9] Chris Iliades, M.D., "Is Juicing Good for Digestive Health?" Viewed online at http://www.everydayhealth.com/digestive-health/is-juicing-good-for-digestive-health.aspx on 10.03.12.

[10] Ibid.

[11] Jennifer K. Nelson, R.D., L.D., "Is Juicing Healthier than Eating Whole Fruits or Vegetables?" Viewed online at http://www.mayoclinic.com/health/juicing/AN02107 on 10.03.12.

[12] Mayo Clinic Staff, "Dietary Fiber: Essential for a Healthy Diet." Viewed online at http://www.mayoclinic.com/health/fiber/NU00033 on 10.03.12.

[13] "Health Benefits of Fruit and Vegetable Juice." Viewed online at http://www.joybauer.com/food-articles/fruit-and-vegetable-juice.aspx on 10.03.12.

[14] Ibid.

[15] Chris Iliades, M.D., "Is Juicing Good for Digestive Health?" Viewed online at http://www.everydayhealth.com/digestive-health/is-juicing-good-for-digestive-health.aspx on 10.03.12.

[16] Winston Craig, MPH, PhD, RD, "Health Benefits of Vegetarian Diets." Viewed online at http://www.vegetarian-nutrition.info/updates/vegetarian_diets_health_benefits.php on 10.03.12.

[17] "The Barriers to Vegetable Consumption." Viewed online at http://www.campbellnutrition.com/VegetablesAndFruits/VegetableConsumption/ on 10.03.12.

[18] "Processed vs. Natural Juices." Viewed online at http://www.discountjuicers.com/naturaljuices.html on 10.03.12.

[19] Robert St. John, "Freshly Squeezed Orange Juice," September 17, 2012. Viewed online at http://robertstjohn.com/2012/09/17/freshly-squeezed-orange-juice/ on 10.03.12.

[20] "Processed vs. Natural Juices." Viewed online at http://www.discountjuicers.com/naturaljuices.html on 10.03.12.

[21] Ibid.

[22] Ibid.

[23] Ibid.

[24] Maria Blanco, "How to Properly Break a Detoxing Juice Fast," Sept. 17, 2009. Viewed online at http://suite101.com/article/how-to-properly-break-a-detoxing-juice-fast-a149421 on 10.01.12.

www.ingramcontent.com/pod-product-compliance
Lightning Source LLC
Chambersburg PA
CBHW060230290526
45789CB00003B/1493